Disclaimer

This book is intended for educational use only. The author holds no responsibility/liability for how the information is used. Whilst this book has been thoroughly researched it does not replace the advice of a trained nutritionist, psychologist, physician or any other professional. Please seek a professional opinion before changing your diet, lifestyle or any other aspect.

My Story

I'll keep this bit short and sweet so you can get to the good bit. I have written this book to help others who struggle with binge eating, as I once did. The journey often felt long and never ending so I wanted to provide others the fast route to giving up this bad habit. This book will help you remove some of the trial and errors associated with binge eating.

Contents

`

Binge Eating Defined

It starts off small. Maybe just one cupcake. Then, before you realize what happened, the entire dozen is gone. All that is left is a little frosting to show that they were even there. How much time has passed? Not long at all – about ten minutes. How is that possible? The more you think about what just happened, what you ate, and how quickly you ate, the more you begin to talk down to yourself. You're angry. "I am terrible. Why couldn't I stop?" You're upset. "What's wrong with me?"

If you have experienced anything like this, the likelihood is you were binge eating. Engaging in binge eating doesn't mean you're a terrible person; it means there was an emotional or physical void that needed to be filled.

Binge eating involves uncontrollable consumption of food during a short time frame. This results in feelings of physical discomfort and pain, as well as feelings of anger, depression, and anxiety[1,2]. It doesn't matter if you weren't hungry to begin with, or you feel full whilst binging, you just feel compelled to carry on.

Binge eating can affect anyone, of any age; although, females are more likely than males to be effected. Individuals normally develop such behaviors during their late teens or early 20s[1]; however, this does not mean that binge eating cannot begin in childhood or in later adulthood. In fact, in the United States, more than 2% of adults experience this problem[2]. This equates to around 4 million adults in the US, not to mention the rest of the world.

Binge eating starts for a variety of reasons. It is not a conscious behavior, you probably didn't wake up thinking "I'm going to eat so much today that I feel horrible both physically and emotionally." No. Instead, it is likely that many different factors contributed to you binge eating, including:

- **Skipping meals** – Regardless of why you skipped a meal, either because you didn't have the opportunity to eat or chose not to, this can lead to binge eating. Your body requires a certain amount of fuel to function effectively, when this threshold isn't reached, your body will feel like it needs more food than necessary. This is a primal reaction to survive when food resources are low.

- **Inability to deal with emotions** – Experiences can cause extreme stress. Often in times of emotion we do not know what actions to take especially when this is a prolonged emotion such as stress. In such situations we tend to cover our feelings using a mask of fat and sugar which helps dampen down the nerves for a short amount of time, allowing our mind to rest.

- **Genetics** – There is some evidence to suggest a link between genes and binge eating due to the problem occurring within families[2]; however this could be a learnt behavior and not fully explained by genetics alone.

- **Depression** – Depression can cause a person to eat as a way to feel better. At least 50% of those who binge eat either have, or have experienced, depression[2].

How many of the factors do you relate too? Using the four bullet points as a start, write down everything you think has contributed towards your binge eating. Many of you will find that the onset of binging was caused by stress, depression or anxiety and research has backed this up, so don't worry you are not alone[1,2,3].Researchers also agree that binge eating has at least one certain outcome, and that is weight gain[1,2]. Due to the detrimental effect that this causes, learning how to stop binge eating is essential.

Health Problems Associated with Binge Eating

The longer it goes on, the worse it gets. You start noticing your clothes fitting tighter. You've gained a few pounds here and there, so that's not too bad, right? You think to yourself, It's okay; you will lose it soon enough. You plan to skip breakfast, and maybe lunch, because who needs those meals anyway? But then reality strikes and by dinner time you're starving. You need something quick and easy because you feel shaky and weak. That family-size bag of chips looks far too good to resist. It couldn't hurt, right? After all, you missed breakfast and lunch. You sit there munching, while watching your favorite show. You feel so much better now and will worry about losing the weight tomorrow or maybe you'll start on Monday.

A lot of us think like this. I know I have.

You might think skipping meals will help you lose weight, but in reality, this actually could be the cause of binge eating[2]. Think about it like this. How many calories are in a family-size bag of chips? About 150 calories per serving. That's not bad, but that's ONE serving. After skipping a meal you think you can justify the whole bag, but each pack contains between 11 and 17 servings ranging from 1650 to 2550 calories. Yikes! That is the daily recommended calories wiped out. Eating that in one sitting, and eating other foods, such as cookies, sandwiches, or cupcakes just adds more calories. It's no wonder we gain weight. You might be a normal weight right now, but what will adding a pound a week do? That's more than 50 pounds in a year. What could that do to your body?

It is the beginning of problems that may lay hidden for a while. These problems aren't associated with the extra money you have to spend to buy larger clothes, although that is a pain. They are rooted in mental and physical issues that are brought about by the weight gain.

Binge eating causes an individual to feel bad about themselves, as well as to have depression and feelings of negativity[4] about how much, and what they ate. Often, these negative feelings lead to us to engaging in this behavior again and again. We create a negative pattern that becomes deep rooted and hard to break.

Feeling bad about yourself, having depression, and feeling guilty is only the beginning. Binge eating can cause multiple physical problems that diminish the quality of life and have the potential to lead to early death. These health problems include:

- **Diabetes** – Obesity is one of the primary contributing factors in the development of type 2 diabetes[5]. Diabetes is one of the top 10 causes of death in the United States. If it doesn't cause death; however, it can cause disfigurement through often needed amputations of the lower limbs (toes, feet, and legs)[6].

- **Heart disease** – Obesity plays a major role in the development of heart disease and subsequent issues with the heart, including heart attack, heart failure, stroke, and arrhythmia[5].

- **High blood pressure** – Obesity causes the heart to beat harder, because more pressure is required to move the blood throughout the body. The risks of high blood pressure include blood clots, stroke, heart damage, kidney damage, memory, vision loss, and damage to the arteries.

- **High cholesterol** – Cholesterol affects the heart. High cholesterol has the potential of blocking arteries and preventing blood flow. This could result in a heart attack, heart failure, or stroke.

- **Asthma** – Obesity can cause asthma. If it does, then it will likely be more severe and more difficult to treat due to bearing extra weight and changes in inflammation[7]. Because of this it is likely that an obese individual with asthma will have a reduced quality of life and may experience distressing episodes of breathlessness.

- **Sleep apnea** – Obesity has been linked to the development of sleep apnea[8]. Not only does sleep apnea make it difficult to get a good night's sleep, it also causes other problems, such as high blood pressure, stroke, and irregularity in the heart beat.

All of these potential physical problems that are associated with obesity are pretty scary. The short term emotions involved in these cycles of binge eating have severe consequences in the long term if not managed correctly. It is important to fully grasp this point and later on in the book I will go through your daily patterns that can help you make those important short term changes to your routine. In the next chapter we will explore the psychology and science behind those short-term thoughts. But if you want to skip to making those changes to your daily routines straight away, take a look at the Step-By-Step guide page.

Emotional Eating: The Psychology and Science Behind Binge Eating

It was one of those days, nothing went right and you still have so much to do. The stress of your responsibilities is starting to get to you and you aren't sure whether to laugh or cry about everything piling up. You just want to be in a better mood. The more you think about everything, the more you realize you need a quick pick-me-up. The cravings have started. You need sugar, and lots of it, but having something salty and crunchy would be great too. Suddenly, you're starving. It's as though you haven't eaten all week. You reach for anything that sounds good that might satisfy these intense cravings. And so it begins…you are now emotional eating.

Emotional eating and binge eating work together. Binge eating can happen at any time, for any reason, but often it is due to emotions[9]. Emotional eating involves unhealthy food choices that we think will make us feel better. However, it causes us to crash and feel horrible both physically and mentally. When we engage in emotional eating, the more we eat, the more we want. This eating pattern becomes difficult to stop as we are not only trying to satiate our food cravings but we are also using it as a tool to change and inhibit certain emotions.

Emotional eating is the result of intense emotions. From the opening scenario, it appears that this only happens when you have a bad day, but this isn't always the case. Emotional eating can happen due to many different situations:

- **Feeling stressed, angry, depressed** – These feelings are common in individuals who emotional eat. We may not consciously intend to over eat. Instead what happens is you feel a void or tension in your body, then you begin to have a craving for something a bit naughty and you can't really focus on anything else. You have to satisfy that craving, knowing that it will help ease the feelings.

- **Wanting to ignore emotions** – Sometimes we just don't want to feel what we're feeling. Maybe we are really upset about a break-up or missing out on that promotion. Drowning ourselves in a huge bag of candy will take our mind off it.

- **Feeling bored**– Boredom is a huge catalyst for binge eating. You know you're not hungry, it's mindless overeating, giving you extra calories that you don't need.

- **Feeling excited, happy, or if you're celebrating** – Emotional eating doesn't have to only be about negative emotions. We also eat when we're happy or excited. How many times have you gone out for food or dessert, because you got a bonus at work, passed your class, or just overall had a good day? You're celebrating, so what does it matter? It matters because you're associating food with reward. Which means when you're having a bad day you're more likely to use food as a pick me up.

Just imagine all those foods you crave when you're having different emotions. What are their primary ingredients? Are they high in fat and sugar?

The high fat foods we crave when experiencing intense emotions are usually processed foods. Foods that are sweet and have a high fat content effect the opioid systems in the brain[10]. The opioid system is extensive throughout the central nervous system, and controls a number of different behaviors such as mood and addiction (including addiction to drugs)[11]. In fact, research has indicated that food cravings, and food addiction, can be similar to drug addiction[12].

When we experience stress, anxiety, or depression, we are also likely to reach for something high in sugar. There are several reasons why sugary foods are appealing. Firstly, the brain uses glucose (a compound which sugar is broken down to) almost exclusively as its energy source. If we have restricted carbohydrates, our brain will not be functioning as effectively. Similarly to high fat sweet foods, high sugar foods hit parts of the brain that are also associated with drug addiction. High sugar foods not only effect the opioid system but also dopamine pathways[13]. Dopamine is known as a 'feel good' chemical in our brains. In animal models binge eating on sugar has led to increased release of dopamine (happy hormone)[14]. These models also become desensitized to the sugar after extended feeding and find it harder to become satiated[15]. Much in the same way that a drug user needs more and more to get a high each time. Furthermore there is evidence to suggest that a diet high in sugar can affect the structure of some cells in the brain[16]. Such changes and the 'drug like' behavior of palatable food has also been witnessed on humans by using brain imaging techniques[17].

Not only does sugar effect our brain it can also impact our hormones. Cortisol is a stress hormone and it is a necessary, evolutionary, hormone that helps us prepare to either flee or fight in a dangerous situation. Cortisol is believed to cause a greater desire for food in binge eaters[18]. When we stress our pituitary gland starts pumping out more cortisol. Long term effect of such prolonged stress and cortisol can reap havoc on the body including effects on the immune system, depression, mood and weight[19]. Your body is looking for a way to reduce stress and find balance. A fast way to do this is by consuming sugar which has been shown to reduce cortisol levels. Sweeteners do not have the same stress reducing impact as sugar, so it's time to put the fizzy drinks down too[20]. Better ways to reduce cortisol are to have a healthy diet, to exercise and to meditate.

Eating sugary foods causes high amounts of glucose leading us to the infamous sugar high. However, the crash soon follows as insulin kicks in and the body starts taking glucose up into cells. To compensate for the crash in blood sugar our body tells us we are hungry and need something sweet. This leads to a vicious cycle of cravings.

Getting caught in the trap of emotional eating can be detrimental to our health and well-being. For this reason, we have to figure out if we are eating because we are emotional, or if we are genuinely hungry. The differences between emotional hunger and physical hunger are as follows:

Emotional Hunger:	**Physical Hunger**:
Happens suddenly	Happens gradually
Desperate need for food satisfaction while	Eating can wait for a
Specific food cravings will be good	No cravings, anything
Is insatiable goes away	When you're full, it
Can't stop thinking about food felt is the stomach	No thoughts of food, is
Feelings of guilt and shame afterwards negative feelings	Does not trigger any

These distinctions are very important, because it's possible that the hunger you're feeling is emotional, rather than physical. The only way to be certain which it is, is to wait. To ensure that you're not bored or emotional, do an activity: go for a walk, play with a pet, or talk on the phone. If you're still hungry after this, the likelihood is that you're experiencing physical, rather than emotional hunger.

Research indicates that felt emotions, such as sadness, anger, and depression, are not the only precursors to emotional eating, or binge eating. In fact, sometimes just the perceived threat of an emotion could lead to emotional eating[21]. For example, imagine you have a presentational job interview next week, the thought is enough to cause us stress even though we are not currently experiencing the situation. It's also possible that being around somebody who is experiencing an emotional state could impact you as well.

Often those who are most affected by other people's emotions are not able to express their own feelings in a constructive way[21]. Being apathetic, hiding and ignoring emotions has a way of coming back to bite us. The extent to which you are able to understand and manage emotion makes up your level of emotional intelligence.

Emotional intelligence helps us not only understand our own emotions, but also the emotions of those around us. This allows us to filter other people's emotions stopping them overtaking our own. Increasing your general self awareness and emotional intelligence will allow you to identify what is causing bad decision making. For example knowing that when you are feeling sad you reach for the ice cream.

If you think you might have trouble getting a handle on your emotions, you're not alone. A lot of people are unsure exactly how to express themselves. This could be due to culture, upbringing, or even gender. The good thing is that you can learn how to manage your emotions, doing so will allow you to gain back control of your emotional eating.

A few ways to handle your feelings include:

- **Learn your triggers** – Triggers happen all the time. It is often difficult to escape them. What is important is learning what those triggers are. If a certain individual makes you angry they are the trigger. Learn to handle the situation better or avoid where possible to remove the negative feelings which could potentially cause a binge.

- **Question what you're doing** – If you don't know why you're feeling or acting a certain way, get some quiet time and try to figure it out. How many times have you said, "I don't know why I'm eating, I'm not even hungry"? If you ever say this to yourself, take a step back and try to figure out how you got to this point. Sometimes discussing this with someone is good and other times just writing stuff down and trying to figure out what is going on can be very beneficial.

- **Examine the big picture** – Are your emotions the result of something bigger? For example is there an experience from your childhood that still floods your mind today or a bad decision that you have made that you have not forgiven yourself for yet.

We have now discussed what binge eating is and where the problems lie. As you can now tell it will include overcoming physical, emotional and mental challenges. By leveraging the knowledge of health problems associated with binge eating you will be able to reach your goal. This new life will provide you with greater energy, a better outlook and a sense of achievement.

How to enjoy food the right way

As with overcoming most obstacles the mind is the first place to start. If you get your head in the game and break down your own barriers and beliefs you can conquer anything, including binge eating. Your mind is your most important asset, how you see and view food will establish and determine the sort of relationship you have with it. Through this chapter I want to guide your mind into the right way of looking at food. Focusing on how you can look internally to identify and specifically eliminate the target thus clamping down on over eating and the inevitable weight gain.

We all look at ourselves differently and we usually judge ourselves harder than we judge others. We even jump to conclusions about our own identity which can leave us in a box and playing the role of someone we ourselves wouldn't aspire to be. This sort of thinking plays a part in why we binge eat. Do you label yourself as a 'binge eater' or even as 'fat' or 'useless'? Do you think it's just who you are and how you cope with situations? Maybe you think you are just not strong enough to kick a habit like this, especially when the cravings start kicking in. Well, your mind is a powerful tool and the way you think will be the way you act. You need to change your narrative and understand that you have overcome obstacles before and you can overcome them again. Think of how you felt when you achieved that promotion, that grade, or that win, you feel pretty impressed with yourself, right? That is also who you are, you are strong, determined and gifted. What we think brings us certain emotions, certain emotions make us binge. By identifying your emotions and triggers you can eliminate negative thought patterns and consciously switch them for a more positive way of thinking. This will create clearer paths to help reach your goals faster. The difference will be felt both physically and mentally.

It's not just the way you look at yourself, it's the way you look at food. Often when we feel tired we will look at high sugary foods and think "that will give me the energy I need", more than say a piece of fruit. Lets test this belief. When we eat the sugar laden food, we get the high which makes us feel good but the crash soon follows and we feel even more sluggish. So short term good, long term bad. A piece of fruit on the other hand will give you a bit of sugar rush but the fibre in it will stop the crash being so hard and help to prolong your energy.

Maybe you don't eat food for the energy but rather to fill a void, to dampen stress or anxiety. Emotional eating is a short term fix for a long term problem. Eating this way will make you feel worse, particularly when your belly is at full stretch. You're bloated and now also suffering from guilt for letting yourself down again. It doesn't have to be like this, just a little reprogramming of the brain needs to happen. Don't use food to handle your emotions, instead face them head on. Hunger is a physical need, thoughts and emotions are not. If you're feeling down ask yourself why, try and change your circumstances so you reduce the emotion particularly if it comes up time and time again. Start thinking of food as fuel and as nourishment. Be aware of how much physical activity your doing and try and eat in proportion to that rather than using it to get quick fixes. Another way is to try and keep your glucose and insulin levels stable by eating high glycaemic foods such as wholemeal bread, legumes and sweet potatoes.

Not only is it important to listen to your mind and navigate your thoughts but it also vital to listen to the signals in your body. Firstly, when our bodies are craving something it means we are deficient and your yearnings are directing you straight in the wrong direction, perhaps the cookie jar. However, if you look at the table below you can see that you can get what your body needs using healthy foods that aren't going to expand your waistline and that you can add into numerous snacks and healthy recipes. You need to predetermine in your mind that you are going to choose the healthy snack and to listen to your body before it actually happens. This way you are helping to reprogram your brain and aren't just relying on your willpower in that moment of weakness.

Craving	Nutrient deficiency	Alternative options
Fatty food	Calcium	Watercress, low fat cheese and milk, broccoli, almonds, sardines
Carbs (bread, pasta etc)	Nitrogen	Beef, chicken, turkey, sardines, shrimp, lobster, cauliflower, spinach, asparagus, eggs
Soda	Calcium	Watercress, low fat yoghurt, broccoli, almonds, sardines
Chocolate	Magnesium	Spinach, pumpkin seeds, mackerel, brown rice, avocados, bananas
Salty foods	Sodium Chloride	Raw sea salt, tomatoes, lettuce and olives
Sugary foods and sweets	Chromium Phosphorus	Mushrooms, kidney beans, pomegranate and pineapple Pumpkin seeds, salmon, tuna, brazil

	Tryptophan	nuts, lentils
	Sulphur	Pumpkin seeds, cheese, beef, chicken, tuna, oats, white beans, eggs
		Eggs, onions, cabbage, broccoli, watercress

Whilst your body may be lacking in a certain vitamin or mineral. You may in fact just be dehydrated and the signal is being confused for hunger so make sure you are drinking plenty of water, at least half your body weight in fluid ounces gives you a good estimate.

A common side effect with binge eating is the increased speed of consumption. You may notice that when your binge eating, you're at top speed. Food goes in, you chew just enough so that you can swallow, then you grab the next bite. This is probably one of the worst habits we have as binge eaters. The signals from our stomach can be a little slow at travelling to the brain. Often the signal of feeling full arrives at the brain 20 minutes later.. so you were full 20 mins ago! At the pace you eat when bingeing, you're not consciously acknowledging the amount food being consumed, how it smells, looks or tastes and you miss the feeling of satiation.

This however can simply be rectified by eating slower and removing any distractions from the environment so you can fully focus on the food. Particularly with the 'bad' food, take time to enjoy it, smell it, take one bite and make that bite last. Really taste the food. After doing this you may feel you don't need half as much as you thought you did. Put your mind in your stomach. How is your stomach feeling? Is it feeling full, how stretched is it? Eat until the feeling of hunger has just gone otherwise this may lead to weight gain. Remember you do not have to finish your plate (even when attending a dinner party) and you do not have to finish a packet. Your body is the priority, not finishing what's in front of you.

Getting to know portion sizes is important and finding out what size works for you. A number of things can lead to a binge. One of these factors maybe not eating enough or skipping meals... like breakfast? Firstly letting yourself get into a state of starvation is detrimental as you will eat far more than if you are keeping topped up with healthy snacks throughout the day. Secondly, breakfast as you know is the most important meal of the day. It kick-starts your metabolism and breaks the fast of the night. We want to avoid our body going into starvation mode as it means we are going to pack more weight on later when we do eat. Therefore ensure you have enough time to enjoy a nutritious breakfast and prepare snacks for between meals such as fruits and nuts.
Meal times should also consist of the right amount of vegetables, protein fat and carbohydrates as this will stop your cravings due to deficiencies or lack of energy.

A simple routine to keep your body working optimally is to snack between meals. I find that having breakfast, snack, lunch, snack and dinner works well. I have listed some snacks below to give you an idea of some healthier alternative for between meals.

Healthy snacks:

- almonds
- bananas
- fruit smoothie
- vegetable juices
- carrot sticks dipped in humus

Top tip: *Another little trick that helps to curb appetite and promote weight reduction is to eat medium chain triglycerides[22]. Eating a teaspoon full of coconut oil or adding it into your coffee should help to curve them afternoon cravings.*

You need to predetermine in your mind that you are going to choose the healthy snack and to listen to your body before it actually happens. This way you are helping to reprogram your brain and aren't just relying on your willpower in that moment of weakness.

Step by step guide

In the following section of the book the key factors and steps that are required for giving up binge eating will be defined in detail to help you reach your goals. Each step will be explained so you can start an actionable plan. At the end there will be a cheat sheet you can look at for quickness. It's a good idea to stick it on your fridge or cupboard to help you get back on track when the cravings start rearing their ugly heads.

Define your goal

It is really important when making changes that you have something to measure. This allows you to see your progress and track how well you are doing. Think of it like an Olympic athlete training for their 100m run without a stopwatch. It acts as a feedback so that if something isn't working for you, you can adjust and change it. With binge eating you need to decide where you're currently at and where you want to go, both in the short and long term. Of course, you eventually want to give up binge eating completely, but it's a good idea to have short to medium length goals as they are more reachable and more motivating. As soon as you hit them you will gain the momentum to give up completely.

So how do we track binge eating? Binges can be defined as either moderate or severe. A moderate binge consists of eating 2-4 'bad snacks'. A full out binge consists of 5 or more. You can track what types of binges you have using this chart.

	Mon	Tue	Wed	Thu	Fri	Sat	Sun
No Binge							

Moderate Binge						
Excessive binge						

Once this has been determined set your goals as below.

How many times are you binge eating in a week/month (fill out the below)?

Current Goal: Number of moderates-   Number of severe-

Medium Goal: Number of moderates-   Number of severe-

End Goal: Number of moderates-   Number of severe-

This is the same for if you are losing weight and the two goals will coincide.

How much do you weigh?

Current:
Medium Goal:
End Goal:

It is really important to see these goals as a scale. You will start off at the beginning and you will be moving forward along the scale, even if you haven't reached your midterm goal yet you're still progressing. If you find it more motivating break the steps down even further. It is important to do what best works for you.

Identify your triggers

There is always a reason for why we binge even if we don't feel like there is. It is really important to identify the pattern that is leading to your bad habit so you can change what is going on. If you are struggling to see what is setting you off, start daily journaling. List what has happened to you in the day, how it made you feel and what foods you ate. I have outlined some common triggers below to help you get started.

- Feeling overwhelmed
- Stress at work
- Stress at home
- Not eating enough food
- Anxiety
- Painful experiences that happened in the past
- Low self esteem
- Boredom

Once you have identified the causation, there may be several factors, ask yourself how can you reduce the influence of these aspects. For each trigger come up with as many ways as possible to eliminate them, then pick the top 2 or 3 that would be most effective.

Trigger: _____

1. _____
2. _____
3. _____

Trigger: _____

1. _____

2. _____
3. _____

Remove all triggers and binge foods

This is a simple but very effective step. Go into your kitchen and throw out all the food that you binge on, this will mainly be the 'junk' food that your body craves. Firstly, you simply cannot binge on it if it's not in the cupboard but secondly, as it's not there for a quick comfort fix you will have to find an alternative method to make yourself feel better. My advice would be to change your environment or mix up your routine. For example go for walk, play with your kids or do some gardening. If you're feeling stressed and your chest is feeling tight have a bath or try doing some meditation or yoga to calm down and relax.

Talk it out

One of the main triggers for binge eating is emotion that has built up without being faced head on. Often we hide things away, maybe we don't want other people to know we are having a difficult time, or maybe we don't want to be honest with ourselves. These thoughts and emotions may bubble a way under the surface for a while and then lead to comfort eating to help fill the hole. This emotion leads us to a behaviour that does not serve us positively. Therefore such emotions must be dealt with differently. One way in which to do this is to talk them out. It is important do this with someone who is neutral, who will not judge you and will allow you to speak honestly. It may surprise you what you have been hiding away. If you feel you do not have a family member or a friend you would feel completely at ease with, do not feel embarrassed or ashamed to seek out a professional. In the end you will feel a weight has been lifted off your shoulders. Our minds can be a cruel place often exaggerating emotions making past or future experiences look far worse than they actually are. Talking helps to put everything into perspective and it could be the single most important thing you do.

Visualisation and preparation

The key to any success lies within your own mind and it is the first place you should prepare for the battles of emotional hunger and cravings. To begin with, you must believe you can give up binge eating... and of cause you can! You have more than likely faced more difficult challenges in your life and come out fighting. Think of three times where you have faced a challenge and overcame it. List them below.

-
-
-

Whenever you feel under confident in your ability to achieve, come back to these bullet points.

Next we must prepare for the challenges that are going to arise. Each night think about what is planned for the following day both at work and at home. If there is a situation that is likely to put you in a bad state and lead to binging think about how you could either completely remove it or reduce its impact on your emotions. Ask yourself how can I make this situation better? After doing this, imagine yourself eating only healthy, wholesome and nutritious foods and saying no to 'junk' food. It is good practice to make your mind up the night before about how you are going to eat and what foods you will say no too, it means you will rely less on willpower in the moment. Go through the same thought process when you wake up in the morning to imprint it into your mind for the day. In addition, start identifying yourself as healthy and confident; ditch the negative labels. Here are some good affirmations to repeat to yourself to help you start your day the right way. Feel free to come up with others if the following do not resonate with you.

- *Today I am going to eat clean*
- *I am healthier now than I have ever been*
- *I am confident in my body*

Make a weekly meal plan

The next stage is to complete a weekly meal plan. Draw on a piece of paper 8 columns split into 6 rows, as below.

	Monday	Tuesday	Wednesday	Thursday	Friday	Saturday	Sunday
Breakfast							
Snack 1							
Lunch							
Snack 2							
Dinner							

Fill in the spaces with healthy wholesome foods that will satisfy you. Have a look at the nutrient deficiencies table in the previous chapter and try and incorporate some of those foods to help curb your cravings for the specific food products. A way to make this table simpler is to have the same breakfast and lunch throughout the week and interchange your snacks and dinner so you don't get bored. The benefit of including snacks amongst your meals is you will never feel hungry and this will keep your metabolism at a high rate.

It is really important that you do a bit of your own research into a healthy diet so you can start planning healthy meals. Stick to simple foods that have minimum ingredients, if the food label sounds like a chemistry master class do not put it into your system. You need to take care of your body as you cannot replace it. Stick to ingredients that have one component i.e. lean meat, fruit and vegetables. Also stick to wholegrain, complex carbohydrates and fats from natural sources such as eggs, salmon and avocado. Learn to make healthy alternatives to your favourite foods, there are tons of recipes to be found on the internet.

It is also important to stick to the correct proportions of food. When serving protein or carbohydrates dish out only a portion that is the size of your fist and then fill the rest of your plate with as many veggies as you want. If you are having a lasagne for example only cut out a piece that is as big as the palm of your hand. It is easy to overeat as you just want to finish what is on your plate. Always serve out a small portion and if you are still hungry serve a little more later.

You may also want to schedule in some meal preparation into the week. This is an excellent idea for example if you always skip breakfast or don't have time to make dinner. Meal preparation involves preparing and making a batch of meals ahead of time so you can just reheat and eat when needed. This not only helps if you are low on time but also with portion size as you can predetermine them in advance and section them out into plastic containers.

This will take up a bit of your time to organise especially in the beginning, but it will get easier and you can always reuse the meal plans you have made. Some of the benefits of meal planning include:

- **Save money**- you will not be buying food that is not needed and ends up in the trash

- **Save time** (in long term)- as you can meal prep in advance

- **Less likely to impulse eat on 'junk'**- as you will already have an alternative healthy option available

- **Save energy**- as you will not need to think of what to have for dinner every nigh

One more key to this component is to ensure you are drinking enough water as dehydration can easily be confused as hunger. Aim to drink at least70.39 fluid ounces a day.

Listen to your body

Your body has built in feedback systems stop overriding them and start listening. Think about when you are binge eating. Where are you, in your head or your belly? Where do you end up in your head or your belly? If you're anything like me, you are mulling over your thoughts that lead to the intense craving at the back of your tongue. You begin cramming thousands of calories worth of food like there is going to be a famine tomorrow. You hardly notice what you're backing in until you stop. Once the episode is over, all you can think about is how big your stomach feels, how much the skin is stretching around your abdomen to compensate for the extra inches you have gained in the past twenty minutes. Not only that but you feel gassy and even a little sick. Your then back in your head beating yourself up about how you have let yourself down again. Well it doesn't have to be this way we just have to pick up the body's signals earlier and begin to act sooner. Move yourself from your head to your gut. Before you even start eating ask yourself is this emotional hunger or am I physically hungry (see previous chapter). If you feel as though your physically hungry have a glass of water and see if it was just dehydration. If you still feel hungry grab a bite to eat. When you do decide to eat sit down remove all distractions and take your time. Keep referring back your stomach and ask how full am I? Am I satisfied? You want to stop as you just start to feel full. As you eat your stomach begins to stretch and sends signals to the brain letting it know you are eating. Listen to these signals and stop appropriately. If you ingest too much food not only will you put on weight but you will feel sluggish due to the energy demand of having to digest it. Small and often is the way to go.

If you feel that you are emotionally hungry do not give into these cravings. If you do, you could potentially feel much worse and this process is about making you feel better. It is really important to do something that you enjoy and increase your dopamine (the happy hormone). Here are a number of ways to increase your dopamine levels naturally:

- meditation[23]
- massage[24]
- sex[25]

Or if none of these suit you have a dance, play your favourite game or listen to some of your music. Put things into perspective and see them for what they are and see your ability to change your situation and your emotions.

Build momentum
In time this process will get easier it will become a natural way of thinking. It's all about putting the effort in now so you can yield the results later. You want to aim to get to a point where you eat only to fuel your body rather than add fire to your emotions. Be able to say no to junk food and be able to have a treat without spiralling into a rampage of eating. To achieve anything worthwhile you will face challenges, difficulties and setbacks but understand that this is a journey and you will become healthier and happier as a result.

Every decision you make you will begin to strengthen new circuits in your brain to form better habits and you will weaken the architecture of you old bad decision making. You have already taken the first few steps on your path to giving up binge eating, you have already bought this book and your this far through. It's time to kick into action and start actioning the steps laid out in this chapter. To make the process even easier follow the cheat sheet below.

Step	Action
1	Define goal
2	Find your triggers and remove them
3	Throw out junk
4	Discuss emotions
5	Visualise success
6	Repeat affirmations
7	Plan food for the week
8	Listen to signals from your body
9	Achieve

Action plan for a relapse

This section is your last resort. I recommend you do not plan for a relapse and understand this might not happen once you have identified your triggers and changed your habits. However, if you do lose yourself, this chapter will help you regain your focus, goals and get you back on your journey to giving up binging and losing weight for good.

1) Don't beat yourself up

So you've just binged, you're probably not feeling great physically and your mind is telling you how stupid you are, or maybe how guilty you should feel. We need to lean away from such thoughts and get into a place of understanding. Relapse is part of your journey, something somewhere has not been effective and changes need to be made so it does not happen again in the future. See this as a feedback mechanism. Look at your chart and look for the positives, maybe this was only a moderate binge compared to what you were doing before or maybe the number of binges has reduced overall for you. This is one episode forgive yourself and move on. You're only being so hard on yourself because of where you want to be physically and emotionally. Take your negative after reaction and use these feelings to motivate yourself not to do this again.

2) Drink water

The next step is to drink water. If you are at full to bursting, just take sips until the food has gone down. Not only will water aid with digestion but being hydrated can also increase your metabolism by up to 30%[26], thus helping to burn through more calories. If you want to go the extra mile add in some lemon/lime not only will it taste better but this will help to increase digestive juices allowing the food to broken down more effectively. As an added bonus these fruits contain citric acid that some suggests can aid weight loss[27].

3) Light exercise

Doing exercise after a binge will make you feel ten times better. It is important to only do light exercising such as walking. The movement will aid digestion so that you get rid of the full sickly feeling faster. It is important that this exercise is kept light, this is not a form of punishment, so I recommend no exercises that get your heart rate through the roof as this will probably make you feel worse. We need to keep most of the blood in the digestive tract instead of dispersed in the muscles. Whilst doing these exercises focus on the benefit it is having on your body, well being and digestion.

4) Refocus

So it is easy once the damage is done to just give up and focus on the negatives. However it is really important to use your actions and emotions at this point to strive towards giving up this bad habit for good. Focus on your goals. Think about what you want your body to look and feel like. Focus on the foods you need to eat to have energy and most importantly focus on succeeding.

5) Analyse

The next step is to analyse what went wrong. There is always a reason or multiple factors that lead to a binge. It may not just be the events that occurred within the day but emotion that has been building for weeks. Have a look back at the triggers you wrote down earlier in the book. Did one of these cause it? Or was it something else? Ask yourself how would you prevent this from happening again?

Your binging behaviour is flagging to you that something is out of balance whether that be physical or emotional. Use this opportunity to put it right so it doesn't keep coming up in the future.

6) Do not skip meals

So after a binge you're feeling excessively full. You have worked out you have surpassed your normal daily calorie limit. You may think, ok, I will just skip breakfast tomorrow or diner later on to lessen the damage. This often does more harm than good not only does it put your body into a state of starvation where it will hold onto more fat, it puts you in the mind set of restriction. The more you restrict the more you will be thinking about foods that you can't eat and the more you are likely to binge. If I said don't think about donuts, what is the first thing you think of? Exactly, never cut out meals or foods as you will be setting yourself up for another episode. If you do still feel over full or not hungry just have a light meal to keep your metabolism burning.

Last Thoughts

You are now on your way to success, you have made it to the end of the book, but this is not the end of the journey, this is just the beginning. Having suffered from binge eating myself for several years, I know how hard the journey to success is. As mentioned previously in the book one of the main keys to success is talking out the problems you experience. Let's face it, nobody is perfect and having the support really helps. Find someone like yourself you can confide in. If you can't think of anyone in your immediate circle checkout Facebook there are loads of supportive groups on there. Good luck with your journey, and just remember persistence and perseverance always pays off.

References

Please note references used were abstract only or open source. Please feel free to continue doing your own research using these as a starting point.

1. Kessler RC, Berglund PA, Chiu WT, Deitz AC, Hudson JI, Shahly V, et al. The prevalence and correlates of binge eating disorder in the World Health Organization World Mental Health Surveys. Biol Psychiatry [Internet]. Elsevier; 2013 May 1 [cited 2016 Oct 6];73(9):904–14. Available from: http://www.ncbi.nlm.nih.gov/pubmed/23290497

2. womenshealth.gov. Binge eating disorder fact sheet | womenshealth.gov [Internet]. Available from: https://www.womenshealth.gov/publications/our-publications/fact-sheet/binge-eating-disorder.html

3. Munn-Chernoff MA, Grant JD, Agrawal A, Koren R, Glowinski AL, Bucholz KK, et al. Are there common familial influences for major depressive disorder and an overeating-binge eating dimension in both European American and African American female twins? Int J Eat Disord [Internet]. 2015 May [cited 2016 Oct 6];48(4):375–82. Available from: http://www.ncbi.nlm.nih.gov/pubmed/24659561

4. Gearhardt AN, White MA, Masheb RM, Morgan PT, Crosby RD, Grilo CM. An examination of the food addiction construct in obese patients with binge eating disorder. Int J Eat Disord [Internet]. Wiley Subscription Services, Inc., A Wiley Company; 2012 Jul [cited 2016 Oct 6];45(5):657–63. Available from: http://doi.wiley.com/10.1002/eat.20957

5. Hinnouho G-M, Czernichow S, Dugravot A, Nabi H, Brunner EJ, Kivimaki M, et al. Metabolically healthy obesity and the risk of cardiovascular disease and type 2 diabetes: the

Whitehall II cohort study. Eur Heart J [Internet]. Oxford University Press; 2015 Mar 1 [cited 2016 Oct 6];36(9):551–9. Available from: http://www.ncbi.nlm.nih.gov/pubmed/24670711

6.   Statistics About Diabetes: American Diabetes Association® [Internet]. Available from: http://www.diabetes.org/diabetes-basics/statistics/?referrer=https://www.google.com/

7.   Dixon AE, Holguin F, Sood A, Salome CM, Pratley RE, Beuther DA, et al. An official American Thoracic Society Workshop report: obesity and asthma. Proc Am Thorac Soc [Internet]. 2010 Sep [cited 2016 Oct 6];7(5):325–35. Available from: http://www.ncbi.nlm.nih.gov/pubmed/20844291

8.   Yu JC, Berger P. Sleep apnea and obesity. S D Med [Internet]. 2011 [cited 2016 Oct 6];Spec No:28–34. Available from: http://www.ncbi.nlm.nih.gov/pubmed/21717814

9.   Macht M. How emotions affect eating: a five-way model. Appetite [Internet]. 2008 Jan [cited 2016 Oct 6];50(1):1–11. Available from: http://www.ncbi.nlm.nih.gov/pubmed/17707947

10. Yanovski S. Sugar and fat: cravings and aversions. J Nutr [Internet]. American Society for Nutrition; 2003 Mar [cited 2016 Oct 6];133(3):835S–837S. Available from: http://www.ncbi.nlm.nih.gov/pubmed/12612163

11. Le Merrer J, Becker JAJ, Befort K, Kieffer BL. Reward processing by the opioid system in the brain. Physiol Rev [Internet]. NIH Public Access; 2009 Oct [cited 2016 Oct 6];89(4):1379–412. Available from: http://www.ncbi.nlm.nih.gov/pubmed/19789384

12. Zhang Y, von Deneen KM, Tian J, Gold MS, Liu Y. Food addiction and neuroimaging. Curr Pharm Des [Internet]. 2011 [cited 2016 Oct 6];17(12):1149–57. Available from: http://www.ncbi.nlm.nih.gov/pubmed/21492080

13. Avena NM, Rada P, Hoebel BG. Evidence for sugar addiction: Behavioral and neurochemical effects of intermittent, excessive sugar intake. Neurosci Biobehav Rev. 2008;32(1):20–39.

14. Avena NM, Rada P, Moise N, Hoebel BG. Sucrose sham feeding on a binge schedule releases accumbens dopamine

repeatedly and eliminates the acetylcholine satiety response. Neuroscience [Internet]. 2006 [cited 2016 Oct 6];139(3):813–20. Available from: http://www.ncbi.nlm.nih.gov/pubmed/16460879

15. Rada P, Avena NM, Hoebel BG. Daily bingeing on sugar repeatedly releases dopamine in the accumbens shell. Neuroscience [Internet]. 2005 [cited 2016 Oct 6];134(3):737–44. Available from: http://www.ncbi.nlm.nih.gov/pubmed/15987666

16. Klenowski PM, Shariff MR, Belmer A, Fogarty MJ, Mu EWH, Bellingham MC, et al. Prolonged Consumption of Sucrose in a Binge-Like Manner, Alters the Morphology of Medium Spiny Neurons in the Nucleus Accumbens Shell. Front Behav Neurosci [Internet]. 2016 [cited 2016 Oct 6];10:54. Available from: http://www.ncbi.nlm.nih.gov/pubmed/27047355

17. Avena NM, Rada P, Hoebel BG. Evidence for sugar addiction: behavioral and neurochemical effects of intermittent, excessive sugar intake. Neurosci Biobehav Rev [Internet]. NIH Public Access; 2008 [cited 2016 Oct 6];32(1):20–39. Available from: http://www.ncbi.nlm.nih.gov/pubmed/17617461

18. Cortisol, Hunger, and Desire to Binge Eat Following a Cold S... : Psychosomatic Medicine [Internet]. Available from: http://journals.lww.com/psychosomaticmedicine/Abstract/2004/11000/Cortisol,_Hunger,_and_Desire_to_Binge_Eat.12.aspx this states

19. mayo clinic. Chronic stress puts your health at risk - Mayo Clinic [Internet]. Available from: http://www.mayoclinic.org/healthy-lifestyle/stress-management/in-depth/stress/art-20046037?pg=2

20. Tryon MS, Stanhope KL, Epel ES, Mason AE, Brown R, Medici V, et al. Excessive Sugar Consumption May Be a Difficult Habit to Break: A View From the Brain and Body. J Clin Endocrinol Metab [Internet]. 2015 Jun [cited 2016 Oct 6];100(6):2239–47. Available from: http://press.endocrine.org/doi/10.1210/jc.2014-4353

21. Fox JRE, Msetfi RM, Johnson RS, Haigh E. The Perception of Threat from Emotions in Predicting Binge Eating

Behaviours in People Who Are Obese and Seeking Treatment for Their Weight. Clin Psychol Psychother [Internet]. 2015 Aug 3 [cited 2016 Oct 6]; Available from: http://www.ncbi.nlm.nih.gov/pubmed/26238312

22. St-Onge M-P, Jones PJH. Physiological effects of medium-chain triglycerides: potential agents in the prevention of obesity. J Nutr [Internet]. 2002 Mar [cited 2016 Oct 6];132(3):329–32. Available from: http://www.ncbi.nlm.nih.gov/pubmed/11880549

23. Kjaer TW, Bertelsen C, Piccini P, Brooks D, Alving J, Lou HC. Increased dopamine tone during meditation-induced change of consciousness. Brain Res Cogn Brain Res [Internet]. 2002 Apr [cited 2016 Oct 6];13(2):255–9. Available from: http://www.ncbi.nlm.nih.gov/pubmed/11958969

24. Field T, Hernandez-Reif M, Diego M, Schanberg S, Kuhn C. Cortisol decreases and serotonin and dopamine increase following massage therapy. Int J Neurosci [Internet]. 2005 Oct [cited 2016 Oct 6];115(10):1397–413. Available from: http://www.ncbi.nlm.nih.gov/pubmed/16162447

25. Damsma G, Pfaus JG, Wenkstern D, Phillips AG, Fibiger HC. Sexual behavior increases dopamine transmission in the nucleus accumbens and striatum of male rats: comparison with novelty and locomotion. Behav Neurosci [Internet]. 1992 Feb [cited 2016 Oct 6];106(1):181–91. Available from: http://www.ncbi.nlm.nih.gov/pubmed/1313243

26. Boschmann M, Steiniger J, Hille U, Tank J, Adams F, Sharma AM, et al. Water-induced thermogenesis. J Clin Endocrinol Metab [Internet]. 2003 Dec [cited 2016 Oct 6];88(12):6015–9. Available from: http://www.ncbi.nlm.nih.gov/pubmed/14671205

27. Mohanapriya M, Ramaswamy L, Rajendran R. HEALTH AND MEDICINAL PROPERTIES OF LEMON (CITRUS LIMONUM). Int J Ayurvedic Herb Med J Homepage [Internet]. 2013 [cited 2016 Oct 6];31095(1). Available from: http://interscience.org.uk/index.php/ijahm

28575700R00023

Printed in Great Britain
by Amazon